I0425001

Recipe Book
for own recipes

Featured images from Pixabay by:
Pettycon

ISBN: 9781093591750

Recipe Name

1 _____
2 _____
3 _____
4 _____
5 _____
6 _____
7 _____
8 _____
9 _____
10 _____
11 _____
12 _____
13 _____
14 _____
15 _____
16 _____
17 _____
18 _____
19 _____
20 _____
21 _____
22 _____
23 _____
24 _____
25 _____
26 _____
27 _____
28 _____
29 _____
30 _____
31 _____
32 _____
33 _____
34 _____
35 _____
36 _____
37 _____
38 _____
39 _____
40 _____

Recipe Name

41 _____

42 _____

43 _____

44 _____

45 _____

46 _____

47 _____

48 _____

49 _____

50 _____

51 _____

52 _____

53 _____

54 _____

55 _____

56 _____

57 _____

58 _____

59 _____

60 _____

61 _____

62 _____

63 _____

64 _____

65 _____

66 _____

67 _____

68 _____

69 _____

70 _____

71 _____

72 _____

73 _____

74 _____

75 _____

76 _____

77 _____

78 _____

79 _____

80 _____

Recipe 1

Servings

_____

Prep Time

_____

Cook Time

_____

Ingredients

_____
_____
_____
_____
_____
_____
_____
_____
_____
_____
_____
_____
_____
_____
_____
_____
_____
_____
_____
_____

Method

_____
_____
_____
_____
_____
_____
_____
_____
_____
_____
_____
_____
_____
_____
_____
_____
_____
_____
_____
_____

Notes

_____

Recipe 2

Servings

Prep Time

Cook Time

_____

_____

_____

Ingredients

Method

Notes

Recipe 3

🥧 Servings

🕐 Prep Time

🕐 Cook Time

🌶 Ingredients

🔪 Method

📝 Notes

Recipe 4

Servings

Prep Time

Cook Time

Ingredients

Method

Notes

Recipe 5

Servings

Prep Time

Cook Time

Ingredients

Method

Notes

Recipe 6

Servings

Prep Time

Cook Time

Ingredients

Method

Notes

Recipe 7

Servings

Prep Time

Cook Time

Ingredients

Method

Notes

Recipe 8

Servings

Prep Time

Cook Time

Ingredients

Method

Notes

Recipe 9

Servings

_____

Prep Time

_____

Cook Time

_____

Ingredients

_____
_____
_____
_____
_____
_____
_____
_____
_____
_____
_____
_____
_____
_____
_____
_____
_____
_____
_____
_____
_____

Method

_____
_____
_____
_____
_____
_____
_____
_____
_____
_____
_____
_____
_____
_____
_____
_____
_____
_____
_____
_____
_____
_____
_____

Notes

_____
_____

Recipe 10

Servings

_____

Prep Time

_____

Cook Time

_____

Ingredients

_____
_____
_____
_____
_____
_____
_____
_____
_____
_____
_____
_____
_____
_____
_____
_____
_____
_____
_____
_____
_____

Method

_____
_____
_____
_____
_____
_____
_____
_____
_____
_____
_____
_____
_____
_____
_____
_____
_____
_____
_____
_____
_____
_____
_____
_____
_____

Notes

_____
_____

Recipe 11

🥧 Servings

🕐 Prep Time

🕐 Cook Time

_____

_____

_____

🌶 Ingredients

🔪 Method

_____
_____
_____
_____
_____
_____
_____
_____
_____
_____
_____
_____
_____
_____
_____
_____
_____
_____
_____

 Notes

_____
_____

Recipe 12

Servings

_____

Prep Time

_____

Cook Time

_____

Ingredients

_____
_____
_____
_____
_____
_____
_____
_____
_____
_____
_____
_____
_____
_____
_____
_____
_____
_____
_____
_____

Method

_____
_____
_____
_____
_____
_____
_____
_____
_____
_____
_____
_____
_____
_____
_____
_____
_____
_____
_____
_____
_____
_____

Notes

_____
_____

Recipe 13

Servings

_____

Prep Time

_____

Cook Time

_____

Ingredients

_____
_____
_____
_____
_____
_____
_____
_____
_____
_____
_____
_____
_____
_____
_____
_____
_____
_____
_____
_____
_____
_____

Method

_____
_____
_____
_____
_____
_____
_____
_____
_____
_____
_____
_____
_____
_____
_____
_____
_____
_____
_____
_____
_____
_____
_____
_____
_____

Notes

_____
_____

Recipe 14

Servings

Prep Time

Cook Time

Ingredients

Method

Notes

Recipe 15

Servings

Prep Time

Cook Time

Ingredients

Method

Notes

Recipe 16

Servings

Prep Time

Cook Time

Ingredients

Method

Notes

Recipe 17

Servings

_____

Prep Time

_____

Cook Time

_____

Ingredients

_____
_____
_____
_____
_____
_____
_____
_____
_____
_____
_____
_____
_____
_____
_____
_____
_____
_____

Method

_____
_____
_____
_____
_____
_____
_____
_____
_____
_____
_____
_____
_____
_____
_____
_____
_____
_____
_____
_____

Notes

_____
_____

Recipe 18

Servings

_____

Prep Time

_____

Cook Time

_____

Ingredients

_____
_____
_____
_____
_____
_____
_____
_____
_____
_____
_____
_____
_____
_____
_____
_____
_____
_____
_____

Method

_____
_____
_____
_____
_____
_____
_____
_____
_____
_____
_____
_____
_____
_____
_____
_____
_____
_____
_____
_____
_____
_____
_____
_____
_____

Notes

_____
_____

Recipe 19

Servings

Prep Time

Cook Time

Ingredients

Method

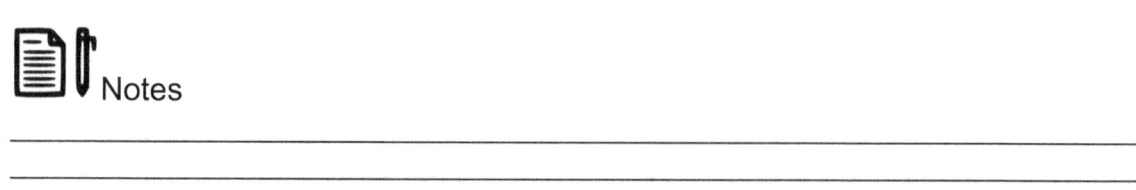

Notes

Recipe 20

Servings

Prep Time

Cook Time

Ingredients

Method

Notes

Recipe 21

Servings

Prep Time

Cook Time

Ingredients

Method

Notes

Recipe 22

Servings

Prep Time

Cook Time

Ingredients

Method

Notes

Recipe 23

Servings

Prep Time

Cook Time

Ingredients

Method

Notes

Recipe 24

Servings

Prep Time

Cook Time

Ingredients

Method

Notes

Recipe 25

Servings

_____

Prep Time

_____

Cook Time

_____

Ingredients

_____
_____
_____
_____
_____
_____
_____
_____
_____
_____
_____
_____
_____
_____
_____
_____
_____
_____
_____
_____

Method

_____
_____
_____
_____
_____
_____
_____
_____
_____
_____
_____
_____
_____
_____
_____
_____
_____
_____
_____
_____
_____
_____

Notes

_____
_____

Recipe 26

Servings
_____

Prep Time
_____

Cook Time
_____

Ingredients
_____
_____
_____
_____
_____
_____
_____
_____
_____
_____
_____
_____
_____
_____
_____
_____
_____
_____
_____
_____

Method
_____
_____
_____
_____
_____
_____
_____
_____
_____
_____
_____
_____
_____
_____
_____
_____
_____
_____
_____
_____
_____
_____

Notes
_____
_____

Recipe 27

Servings

_____

Prep Time

_____

Cook Time

_____

Ingredients

_____
_____
_____
_____
_____
_____
_____
_____
_____
_____
_____
_____
_____
_____
_____
_____
_____
_____
_____
_____

Method

_____
_____
_____
_____
_____
_____
_____
_____
_____
_____
_____
_____
_____
_____
_____
_____
_____
_____
_____
_____
_____
_____

Notes

_____
_____

Recipe 28

Servings

_____

Prep Time

_____

Cook Time

_____

Ingredients

_____
_____
_____
_____
_____
_____
_____
_____
_____
_____
_____
_____
_____
_____
_____
_____
_____
_____
_____
_____

Method

_____
_____
_____
_____
_____
_____
_____
_____
_____
_____
_____
_____
_____
_____
_____
_____
_____
_____
_____
_____
_____
_____
_____

Notes

_____
_____

Recipe 29

Servings

Prep Time

Cook Time

Ingredients

Method

Notes

Recipe 30

Servings

Prep Time

Cook Time

Ingredients

Method

Notes

Recipe 31

Servings

Prep Time

Cook Time

Ingredients

Method

Notes

Recipe 32

Servings

Prep Time

Cook Time

Ingredients

Method

Notes

Recipe 33

Servings

Prep Time

Cook Time

Ingredients

Method

Notes

Recipe 34

Servings

Prep Time

Cook Time

Ingredients

Method

Notes

Recipe 35

Servings

Prep Time

Cook Time

Ingredients

Method

Notes

Recipe 36

Servings

Prep Time

Cook Time

Ingredients

Method

Notes

Recipe 37

Servings

_____

Prep Time

_____

Cook Time

_____

Ingredients

_____
_____
_____
_____
_____
_____
_____
_____
_____
_____
_____
_____
_____
_____
_____
_____
_____
_____
_____
_____
_____

Method

_____
_____
_____
_____
_____
_____
_____
_____
_____
_____
_____
_____
_____
_____
_____
_____
_____
_____
_____
_____
_____
_____
_____

Notes

_____
_____

Recipe 38

Servings

_____

Prep Time

_____

Cook Time

_____

Ingredients

_____
_____
_____
_____
_____
_____
_____
_____
_____
_____
_____
_____
_____
_____
_____
_____
_____
_____
_____
_____

Method

_____
_____
_____
_____
_____
_____
_____
_____
_____
_____
_____
_____
_____
_____
_____
_____
_____
_____
_____
_____
_____
_____
_____
_____

Notes

_____
_____

Recipe 39

Servings

Prep Time

Cook Time

Ingredients

Method

Notes

Recipe 40

Servings

Prep Time

Cook Time

Ingredients

Method

Notes

Recipe 41

Servings

_____

Prep Time

_____

Cook Time

_____

Ingredients

_____
_____
_____
_____
_____
_____
_____
_____
_____
_____
_____
_____
_____
_____
_____
_____
_____
_____
_____

Method

_____
_____
_____
_____
_____
_____
_____
_____
_____
_____
_____
_____
_____
_____
_____
_____
_____
_____

Notes

_____
_____

Recipe 42

Servings
_____

Prep Time
_____

Cook Time
_____

Ingredients
_____
_____
_____
_____
_____
_____
_____
_____
_____
_____
_____
_____
_____
_____
_____
_____
_____
_____
_____

Method
_____
_____
_____
_____
_____
_____
_____
_____
_____
_____
_____
_____
_____
_____
_____
_____
_____
_____
_____
_____
_____
_____
_____

Notes
_____
_____

Recipe 43

Servings

_____

Prep Time

_____

Cook Time

_____

Ingredients

_____
_____
_____
_____
_____
_____
_____
_____
_____
_____
_____
_____
_____
_____
_____
_____
_____
_____

Method

_____
_____
_____
_____
_____
_____
_____
_____
_____
_____
_____
_____
_____
_____
_____
_____
_____
_____
_____
_____
_____
_____

Notes

_____
_____

Recipe 44

Servings

Prep Time

Cook Time

Ingredients

Method

Notes

Recipe 45

Servings

_____

Prep Time

_____

Cook Time

_____

Ingredients

_____
_____
_____
_____
_____
_____
_____
_____
_____
_____
_____
_____
_____
_____
_____
_____
_____
_____
_____
_____
_____

Method

_____
_____
_____
_____
_____
_____
_____
_____
_____
_____
_____
_____
_____
_____
_____
_____
_____
_____
_____

Notes

_____
_____

Recipe 46

Servings

Prep Time

Cook Time

Ingredients

Method

Notes

Recipe 47

Servings

Prep Time

Cook Time

Ingredients

Method

Notes

Recipe 48

Servings

Prep Time

Cook Time

Ingredients

Method

Notes

Recipe 49

Servings

_____

Prep Time

_____

Cook Time

_____

Ingredients

_____
_____
_____
_____
_____
_____
_____
_____
_____
_____
_____
_____
_____
_____
_____
_____
_____
_____
_____
_____

Method

_____
_____
_____
_____
_____
_____
_____
_____
_____
_____
_____
_____
_____
_____
_____
_____
_____
_____
_____
_____

Notes

_____
_____

Recipe 50

Servings

Prep Time

Cook Time

Ingredients

Method

Notes

Recipe 51

Servings

Prep Time

Cook Time

Ingredients

Method

Notes

Recipe 52

Servings

Prep Time

Cook Time

Ingredients

Method

Notes

Recipe 53

Servings

Prep Time

Cook Time

Ingredients

Method

Notes

Recipe 54

Servings

Prep Time

Cook Time

Ingredients

Method

Notes

Recipe 55

Servings

Prep Time

Cook Time

Ingredients

Method

Notes

Recipe 56

Servings

Prep Time

Cook Time

Ingredients

Method

Notes

Recipe 57

Servings

_____

Prep Time

_____

Cook Time

_____

Ingredients

_____
_____
_____
_____
_____
_____
_____
_____
_____
_____
_____
_____
_____
_____
_____
_____
_____
_____
_____
_____
_____

Method

_____
_____
_____
_____
_____
_____
_____
_____
_____
_____
_____
_____
_____
_____
_____
_____
_____
_____
_____
_____

Notes

_____
_____

Recipe 58

Servings

Prep Time

Cook Time

Ingredients

Method

Notes

Recipe 59

Servings

Prep Time

Cook Time

Ingredients

Method

Notes

Recipe 60

Servings

Prep Time

Cook Time

Ingredients

Method

Notes

Recipe 61

Servings

Prep Time

Cook Time

Ingredients

Method

Notes

Recipe 62

Servings

Prep Time

Cook Time

Ingredients

Method

Notes

Recipe 63

Servings

Prep Time

Cook Time

Ingredients

Method

Notes

Recipe 64

Servings

Prep Time

Cook Time

Ingredients

Method

Notes

Recipe 65

Servings

Prep Time

Cook Time

Ingredients

Method

Notes

Recipe 66

Servings

_____

Prep Time

_____

Cook Time

_____

Ingredients

_____
_____
_____
_____
_____
_____
_____
_____
_____
_____
_____
_____
_____
_____
_____
_____
_____
_____
_____
_____

Method

_____
_____
_____
_____
_____
_____
_____
_____
_____
_____
_____
_____
_____
_____
_____
_____
_____
_____
_____
_____
_____
_____
_____

Notes

_____
_____

Recipe 67

Servings

Prep Time

Cook Time

Ingredients

Method

Notes

Recipe 68

Servings

Prep Time

Cook Time

Ingredients

Method

Notes

Recipe 69

Servings

_____

Prep Time

_____

Cook Time

_____

Ingredients

_____
_____
_____
_____
_____
_____
_____
_____
_____
_____
_____
_____
_____
_____
_____
_____
_____
_____
_____

Method

_____
_____
_____
_____
_____
_____
_____
_____
_____
_____
_____
_____
_____
_____
_____
_____
_____
_____
_____
_____
_____

Notes

_____
_____

Recipe 70

Servings

Prep Time

Cook Time

Ingredients

Method

Notes

Recipe 71

Servings

Prep Time

Cook Time

Ingredients

Method

Notes

Recipe 72

Servings

Prep Time

Cook Time

Ingredients

Method

Notes

Recipe 73

Servings

Prep Time

Cook Time

_____

Ingredients

Method

_____

Notes

_____

Recipe 74

🥧 Servings

🕐 Prep Time

🕐 Cook Time

🌶️ Ingredients

🔪 Method

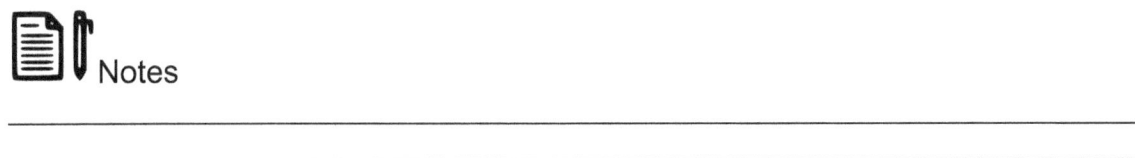 Notes

Recipe 75

Servings

Prep Time

Cook Time

Ingredients

Method

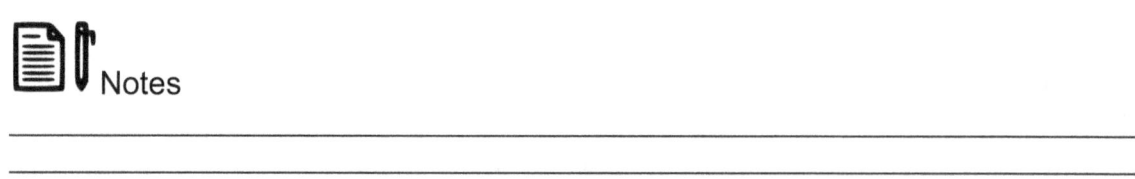

Notes

Recipe 76

Servings

Prep Time

Cook Time

Ingredients

Method

Notes

Recipe 77

Servings

Prep Time

Cook Time

Ingredients

Method

Notes

Recipe 78

Servings
_____

Prep Time
_____

Cook Time
_____

Ingredients
_____
_____
_____
_____
_____
_____
_____
_____
_____
_____
_____
_____
_____
_____
_____
_____
_____
_____
_____
_____

Method
_____
_____
_____
_____
_____
_____
_____
_____
_____
_____
_____
_____
_____
_____
_____
_____
_____
_____
_____
_____
_____
_____
_____

Notes
_____
_____

Recipe 79

Servings

Prep Time

Cook Time

Ingredients

Method

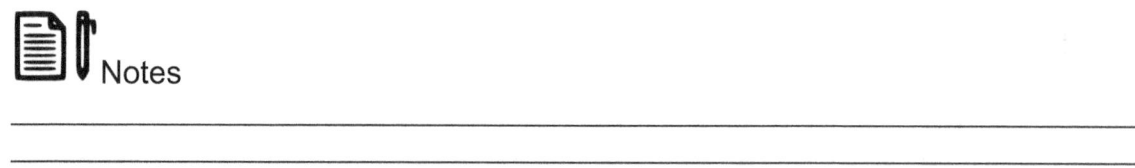

Notes

Recipe 80

Servings

Prep Time

Cook Time

Ingredients

Method

Notes

Quick Cooking Conversions

Volume

1 tablespoon = 3 teaspoons = 15 millilitres
4 tablespoons = 1/4 cup = 60 millilitres
1 ounce = 2 tablespoons = 30 millilitres
1 cup = 8 ounces = 250 millilitres
1 pint = 2 cups = 500 millilitres
1 quart = 4 cups = 950 millilitres
1 quart = 2 pints = 950 millilitres
1 gallon = 4 quarts = 3800 millilitres (3.8 litres)

Temperature

Gas 1 = 275 F = 140 C
Gas 2 = 300 F = 150 C
Gas 3 = 325 F = 170 C
Gas 4 = 350 F = 180 C
Gas 5 = 375 F = 190 C
Gas 6 = 400 F = 200 C
Gas 7 = 425 F = 220 C
Gas 8 = 450 F = 230 C
Gas 9 = 475 F = 240 C

Weight

1 ounce = 28 grams
1000 grams = 1 kilogram
1 kilogram = 2.2 pounds
1 pound = 16 ounces